My experience with Scleroderma

A little known autoimmune disease

Pamela I. Kewin

My experience with Scleroderma, a little known autoimmune disease

Dedicated to Dr. Abdul Rahman Khawaja

Contents

Scleroderma

Scleroderma is an autoimmune, connective tissue disease. The name Scleroderma means hard skin. This is one of the first visible signs of the disease but quite often it takes a few years of suffering till this emerges and it entails much more than this.

It is also named systemic sclerosis.

Scleroderma is a rare disease where the body produces too much collagen which causes the skin thickening. It can cause scarring, disease of the blood vessels and varying degrees of inflammation caused by an overactive immune system. These and other autoimmune diseases occur when the body's tissues are attacked by its own immune system. Medicines like Mycophenolate Mofetil lower the immune system. The formation of scar tissue is called fibrosis; it affects the skin and can affect the internal organs. The involved areas become thick and firm and can cause many problems. Another name for the illness is systemic sclerosis; this is when it is widespread in the body.

There is no cure but there are many treatments which have been found to be effective. Sometimes it is necessary to try various medicines before a suitable one is found and some patients do not need any treatment at all. Others find after a length of time that treatment can be reduced or completely stopped but they will need to be checked on a regular basis.

Quite often a patient might have more than one autoimmune disease at the same time: this is known as an "overlap" illness. It can be that the symptoms of each are milder when they are together than separately, which means that the prognosis is much better.

It is not known exactly why the immune system begins to attack the body but there is constant research into autoimmune diseases and when a cause is found, hopefully soon a cure will also be found.

Who gets Scleroderma?

Scleroderma is more prevalent in women than men. The age when it most commonly develops is between the ages of 35 and 50 but older people and young children can also get it. Young children are more likely to get localised Scleroderma or morphea. This is generally a patch or patches of skin somewhere on the body which do not need treatment but fade in most cases in time. It can be serious so it is important to see a doctor on a regular basis. There are other forms of juvenile Scleroderma which generally do need treatment.

Scleroderma is not contagious and has been believed to be a disease which cannot be inherited but there are some studies of several people in the same family contracting an auto immune illness. This is more often the case if there is a history of rheumatic diseases in the family.

There are a high number of Africans, and again more women, who develop a severe form of Scleroderma compared to the rest of the world and it could be that Scleroderma and auto immune diseases may be hereditary in Africa.

Types of Scleroderma and symptoms

There are two main types of systemic sclerosis: limited cutaneous systemic sclerosis and diffuse cutaneous systemic sclerosis.

In the **limited** form of sclerosis, the skin which is involved is on the fingers, hands, lower arms, lower legs and the face. This used to be referred to as CREST syndrome. CREST stands for: Calcinosis, Raynaud's phenomenon, oesophageal problems, sclerodactyly and telangiectasia. It is now known that these problems also affect patients with diffuse systemic sclerosis so the term CREST is no longer generally used.

In **diffuse** sclerosis the skin involved includes the chest wall and/or all other areas of the body.

Some of the problems that people with systemic sclerosis can face include:

Raynaud's phenomenon: this is a disorder which affects up to 20% of adults worldwide. More women than men are affected and in the UK at least 10% of women suffer from it to some extent.

A Raynaud's attack occurs when the blood flow to the fingers or toes is interrupted. Changes in temperature or stress can be the triggers. The fingers become white and dead-looking, then turn blue and red as the blood begins to flow back. It can be painful with a feeling of numbness or tingling.

Primary Raynaud's occurs with no other condition, most people with this start to experience problems as teenagers, even small children can be affected.

Secondary Raynaud's is usually associated with Scleroderma, Lupus and Rheumatoid Arthritis. It is more problematic than primary Raynaud's as digital ulcers can develop which can become infected and even gangrenous.

Dryness and irritation of the skin and skin ulcers: the most common places to get ulcers are on the fingers and toes, this is why it is very important to try to keep the hands and feet warm. It is when they are white and cold without any feeling for a long time, that they are more susceptible to ulcers. Pitted digital scars are common in systemic sclerosis and have the appearance of an indentation in the skin and may develop into ulcers. Ulcers may also occur on the legs after a knock so care needs to be taken, for example, wearing long trousers rather than shorts or skirts. Leg ulcers on people with Scleroderma take longer to heal and the dressings must be changed several times a week.

On fingers and toes dry dressings are usually sufficient and drugs to help blood circulation may be given. These are called vasodilators and are oral or intravenous. If ulcers become infected it may be necessary to take antibiotics. Eczema can develop around ulcers and steroid creams may be prescribed.

Skin tightening on the face, the fingers and other parts of the body: this is a fundamental problem in Scleroderma. The skin becomes hard and shiny, it is usually itchy and over time it causes contractures or fixed joints. Many people complain that their skin is dry and flaky and often they feel a burning sensation. Over times the skin gets thinner and it needs to be regularly moisturised because the dry skin cracks which is then painful and can become infected. There are various medications which are prescribed for this; exercise and physiotherapy are recommended to keep the skin around the joints flexible. For hands and feet, warm paraffin wax is useful to relax the painful areas, particularly before exercising.

Sclerodactyly: the first signs of this are swollen fingers and hands coupled with shiny, hard skin, also the toes can be affected. After a time it becomes difficult to bend the fingers and as a result of the severe tightening of the skin, they curl and lose mobility, meaning that it is no longer possible to straighten the hands.

Microstomia: this is shrinking of the mouth where the skin on the face and around the mouth becomes hard and tight making it difficult to open the mouth fully. This can seriously affect the teeth as the small mouth opening can makes dental care a problem. The tongue can be affected as well, causing it to lose mobility. A very effective way for a large number of patients with Microstomia to counteract this is to do facial exercises to maintain mobility of the mouth, tongue and face, which can help to stretch the mouth back to its normal or near normal, size.

Telangiectasia: these are small red dots on the face, hands or body. They are dilated blood vessels near the surface of the skin. They can be unsightly and there are laser treatments to remove them.

Calcinosis: calcium under the skin is a complication which some patients develop. It is a chalky material which forms nodules, quite often in the fingers but can occur on any part of the body. It can be hard or semi-liquid and can work its way out of the skin, this sometimes cures the problem but it sometimes becomes ulcerous. Antibiotics may be given or surgery can remove them. This is not always a permanent solution as the nodules often return at the same or new places. Softening the skin with wax can speed up the process of bringing them to the surface.

Digestive problems: in Scleroderma the upper and lower digestive tracts are often affected, with common problems such as acid reflux and swallowing difficulties. Those with swallowing difficulties feel as if the food is stuck in the oesophagus. The oesophagus can shrink and make eating laborious. It is recommended not to lie down for at least an hour after eating. Other symptoms are nausea, vomiting, constipation or diarrhoea, increasing fluid intake, exercising regularly and plenty of fibre in the diet helps.

Heart problems: the heart is one of the major organs affected by Scleroderma. Severe skin tightening can eventually put pressure on all the organs in the body including the heart. Hypertension (high blood pressure) putting strain on the heart is the commonest cause of heart problems.

Lung problems: in Scleroderma there are two ways that the lungs are affected. As with the skin, the membranes which line the lungs can be damaged causing scarring or fibrosis. The second problem is that blood vessels may thicken, narrow and become scarred which may cause pulmonary hypertension. This is often the case about five years after a person develops limited sclerosis. Not everyone will develop lung problems but it is important to test the lungs on a regular basis. There are several tests, the most common being chest X-rays and lung function tests.

Overlap illnesses: in some cases, patients with Scleroderma may have an overlap illness like Polymyositis, which causes inflammation of the muscles. Generally, those with an overlap illness get a milder form of each, in which case they may find that after treatment, their symptoms are not so bad.

It is not usual to get all of these symptoms. Some people are severely affected and others have a very mild form of Scleroderma. It is also sometimes the case that patients suffer for many years of their childhood and later with health problems which are left untreated because their cause is inexplicable. After all kinds of tests no cause can be found for the problems, only to discover in later life that they have had a form of Scleroderma or another autoimmune disease.

The main difficulty diagnosing autoimmune diseases is that the symptoms are like so many other things. Checking for an autoimmune disease seems often to be the last resort after years of suffering in too many cases.

HOW MY SYMPTOMS DEVELOPED

All my life I have been very healthy. In 1989 I moved to Germany and I remember the first year that I lived there I went to the doctor for a general health check. He did various tests including a lung function test. He was very impressed and said my health was more than 100%, better than good. Obviously, nothing can be more than 100%; it was his way of saying that my health was perfect. At the time I was 34 years old.

When I was 37 I had my appendix removed and a few years later I developed an underactive thyroid. I returned to England at the beginning of 2005 and the same year I began to study with the Open University for a degree in English, German and other subjects which took my interest. At the end of 2006 I was working and studying full time. In August of 2007 I went to the Friedrich Schiller University in Jena, East Germany for the summer school for the first year of my German module. I felt tired during and after this time but put it down to the hectic schedule. Our time was filled from early morning to evening with only a break for mealtimes.

After my German exam in October 2007 I had about four months before I started the second year of German so I decided to take two short courses at the same time. They took the whole four months to complete. At the end of this time I was feeling very fatigued but believed it was because of the extra study as well as working.

In 2008 I started my final year of German and felt so exhausted most of the time that I was thinking I would not take my final year of English which began in February 2009. I really did not think I would have the strength. I could have completed my degree without Honours but eventually thought as I had done so much I may as well finish.

9

At the beginning of 2008 I noticed that when I was especially tired my face seemed a different shape and puffy. I was losing weight but it appeared that I had put on weight because my face was fat and puffy and I had developed a double chin.

Whenever I was tired it was worse, I felt that my face was becoming ugly and had no idea why there was such a change.

I began to take all kinds of vitamins and remedies to boost my energy and felt fine for a while. At the beginning of 2009 I was accepted onto a PGCE teacher training course for adult education. A placement could not be found in a school, without which it was not possible to start the course, so I took a preliminary course, Preparing to teach in the Lifelong Learning Sector which I completed in January 2010. I also finished my BA Honours degree and expected that now my studies were finished I would be able to get my energy levels back very soon.

I volunteered for a short time in the local adult education centre and tutored a German girl in English for a few months. I was hoping that I would find a position where I could use my degree.

However, there was no improvement in my health. We had very cold weather at the beginning of 2010 and my hands would go white and numb with cold and as they warmed up I would get a tingling feeling in my fingers which is very painful, that was the beginning of Raynaud's phenomenon which is caused by problems with circulation. I have Secondary Raynaud's which is often one of the first noticeable symptoms of Scleroderma.

Since early 2008 I had noticed stiffness in my knees when I went to stand up after sitting for a while but attributed it to the fact that I stand a lot when I am at work. Slowly over time it became gradually harder to bend my knees. If I crouched down to pick up something, when I stood up it felt as if all the tendons were pulling in my legs. It felt as if they were ripping. It was a very strange and painful feeling. I thought it was work-related and kept searching for a job in the field of work I had thought to enter.

As a result, I did not go to the doctor about this. Around March 2010 I began to notice that when I lay down on my side to sleep, I would get pins and needles in my arms and they would feel numb, I had to struggle to sit up. Then pain in my wrists began and my hands would go numb and tingle if I carried a shopping bag. I researched my symptoms online and found out about Carpal Tunnel Syndrome. I have a friend who is a doctor but he lives in another country so I could not go to see him. I described my symptoms to him and told him what I had found out. He said it is dangerous to try to diagnose my own illness, which I know. I don't make a habit of looking for illnesses. I only put the symptoms I was actually experiencing into Google.

This time I did go to my doctor and he thought it might be Carpal Tunnel Syndrome and made an appointment for me to have tests at the hospital in June 2010. After the tests it was confirmed and the surgeon recommended to my doctor that he first try cortisone injections, which I had at the beginning of July. That was the most painful experience of my life. I nearly passed out and felt very sick, sweat was pouring down my face and the doctor said I had gone puce. The injections did not help at all: in fact the problem was much worse after that. So the decision was made to operate.

The day after I had the cortisone injections I started to get pain in my left leg and a lump appeared on my shin. It felt like a bruise but the lump was white, not discoloured like a bruise. It began to be painful to walk but I thought it would go away soon. About a month later, the same thing started on my right leg. They were both on my shins and over the months walking became very painful and if I stood for a short while then my legs would swell. I went to the doctor and he told me I must have done some excessive exercise but I had not. I had had the pain for so long by then (October) I had forgotten that there was a month between the beginnings of the pain in both my legs. The diagnosis was shin splints (which I later thought could not be right or wouldn't the problem have been in both legs from the beginning?) and to take pain killers and anti-inflammatories. I looked this up on the Internet and found tips for exercises and things to do, like raising my legs and putting icepacks on them. These things did seem to help to some extent but I was also spending a lot of money on painkillers. I kept looking for comfortable shoes and now have enough to last for 10 years at least.

Sometimes if I jolted my legs it felt like an electric shock running through them and I could not take a step. I once had to take a taxi home from the shops and it is only a short walk. Then began the pain in my right instep and I bought all kinds of insoles to support my foot. From this time whenever I walked it felt as if I was walking directly on the bones of my feet. As if there was no shoe on my foot at all.

July 2010 I noticed a triangle of shiny, itchy skin on my chest, just underneath my neck and the same itchiness on my scalp. I was told this was "just cosmetic" and was given various creams and ointments but none helped. Sometimes there was respite from the itchiness, but then it started again. I began to notice with each onset of itching that the patch of skin was growing. I put my symptoms into Google and came up with Scleroderma for the skin and painful joints and also found out information about Myositis, this is inflammation of the muscles, and the description of both matched my symptoms. I kept going to the doctor but did not tell him about my research because I didn't expect him to take what I said seriously. I expected him to criticize me if I mentioned it. Doctors don't expect the patients to visit them with a self-diagnosis. I trusted him but he had no idea what the problem could be. I imagine he put it down to the normal aches and pains that people get as they age.

By the beginning of November I was finding it very difficult to walk, including walking up stairs. At the same time I had my first Carpal Tunnel procedure and had four weeks off work. During this time the pain in my legs improved and I was finding it easier to walk upstairs, but realised that it was because I had been resting. After four weeks my hand was better and almost back to normal and I returned to work at the beginning of December.

The first day at work my left knee suddenly swelled up and from then on I began to feel very unsteady on my feet. My leg would sometimes give way for no apparent reason.

I kept going to the doctor and telling him all the symptoms but he would look at my legs and feet and say he could see nothing and to carry on with the painkillers and see what happens. The only thing that was happening was that my condition was getting worse by the day.

One idea I had was that maybe it was a very severe case of arthritis and a neighbour who is a nurse said the stiffness seemed to point that way. At this time I could not even bend my leg to step onto a curb in the street, even if it was only a couple of inches. I used to see old ladies in their 70's striding along the road and be envious. I really thought it would not be long before I was crippled and not able to walk at all.

I was trying remedies recommended for joint pain like Glucosamine and Chrondotin; I was always searching for something. The best was Litozin which is made from rose hips and was helpful but they are all expensive and not a cure so I stopped taking them. I only took strong painkillers the doctor eventually gave me but nothing took the pain away; it only dulled it for a while. Every day I would use the ice packs. I scoured the Internet for natural remedies as I did not want to rely on painkillers. I only took them if I had to go somewhere or knew I would need to stand for any length of time. I read that dark chocolate is good for arthritic pain and I would buy it and eat a couple of squares a day as recommended. It seemed to help but I think it was more a case of believing it did. I didn't keep it up, it was just a fad.

I noticed at this time that my hands had started to swell and the skin was very shiny and smooth and unless I exercised my fingers, my hands were beginning to stiffen. I would often look at my hands and wonder about it. I was not using my hands very much at the time because they were so painful but could not imagine how that could make the skin shiny. I found it hard to lift my arms above my head and couldn't put them behind my back so getting dressed began to be very difficult. I couldn't pick up even the lightest object and blamed it on the pain; it never occurred to me that it was because I hardly had any strength at this time.

Buttons on clothes felt like knives and I began to wear loose clothes. I couldn't bend my legs to sit down and at home I started to use my office chair pumped up high because it was a strain to stand up. It was as if something was ripping inside my legs every time. If I had an itch on my back the only way to stop it was to rub against a wall. I felt like a bear rubbing against a tree. It is strange how we use animal similes to describe things, because at this time I felt as if I was walking like a penguin, my legs didn't bend at all. I have read comments on forums from people who have said exactly the same thing. It is definitely not as humorous as it sounds.

Just before Christmas 2010, we had snow and I slipped very, very slightly. It was just a slight twist of my left leg but it left me almost crippled for a few days and I was very scared to walk on

14

the snow because of not being able to bend down or stand up from the floor at that time. I thought if I fell in the snow I would not be able to get up and was afraid I would be hit by a car in the middle of the road. I was off work for a week and resting seemed to help.

I had read that riding a bike is good for the knees so I bought an exercise bike and keep it in the living room. In a very short time I began to lose weight rapidly but when I measured my waist or hips there was no change and I wondered where I was losing it from. One day I looked in the mirror and noticed that my arms were withered like an old woman. My thighs were getting thinner too. I was shocked and thought I was aging prematurely. That it was caused by a serious illness did not enter my head.

I knew that there was something wrong with my health but did not know how I could get the doctor to listen. I had lost 5 kilos at this time but never thought that it could all be from my arms and legs or that it could be muscle mass.

Another new symptom at this time was that my mouth appeared to be getting smaller and I had pain and numbness on the right side of my face. In bed at night it would feel as if there was a heater next to my face, it was a very strange sensation. My head felt as if it was stuffed with cotton wool. My jaw hurt, my voice seemed to change and it hurt to talk for long. I couldn't eat properly; I was cutting food small just to get it in my mouth. A visit to the dentist was painful just trying to open my mouth wide enough. The most I could open my mouth was about 30 millimetres.

For several months I had noticed if I lifted anything heavy I would get chest pains and would think I needed to see the doctor about it, but when I stopped and rested I would forget about it because the pain would no longer be there. I also thought it would be a waste of time because of the non-response to the other problems.

As all these health problems came gradually over more than three years I didn't see them as symptoms of one illness. I seemed to be in a daze at this time. I couldn't think straight, everything was pain. The worst thing is that the doctor was taking no notice. Most autoimmune illnesses are not discernible at first and very few doctors know anything about them. All the different symptoms are seen separately and not as part of a whole.

At work if I mentioned pain in my legs, it was just a case of, "women are always complaining of some pain or other." They had no sympathy.

I still kept trying to get something helpful from the doctor but I suppose as my joints were not deformed he could not see what the problem could be. One day I was in the surgery almost in tears, and he said. "You're a crock". This foolish statement did not help at all and it is not something a patient expects to hear from a doctor. During March 2011, I had an appointment for a carpal tunnel operation on the second hand and every day till then was a struggle. From the beginning of the year I had stopped going to the doctor. I was hoping that somehow when I had time off after my operation I would manage to get an answer to my health problems.

By this time I could not do simple tasks like opening a can, (I bought an electric can opener even though I rarely need it) and had to wait for visitors to open bottles. I could no longer get into the bath, and had to hold on to the bannister and drag myself up the stairs to my apartment. I would be in tears with the pain every day when I got home; at the end it was almost impossible to turn the key in the lock to open the door. Every time I had to use my hands it was agony.

I was very scared; I live alone and thought in a very short time I would be crippled. It did not seem possible to me that after all my visits to the doctor I could have all these problems and the doctor did not have a remedy.

By this time I felt that it would not be long before I would need a wheelchair. When I lay down it was almost impossible to turn over from one side to the other. I could not raise my head from the pillow. I used to lie down and try to exercise my legs by raising them up. If I could manage a couple of inches I would feel as if I had achieved something big and hoped it was a sign of recovery.

To sit up in bed, I would have to roll over onto my side, lower my feet to the floor, push myself up and with great agony, stand up, move further up the bed and sit down again. Lifting my legs back onto the bed was an effort, too. I would also go to sleep with my legs straight in bed and hope that while I slept I did not bend my legs. If I woke up and my legs had moved in my sleep, it used to be very painful to straighten them out. It almost felt as if they were locked into position. I used to do exercises every day to try to strengthen my legs and make them more flexible, but I could never feel any benefit.

Because of the pain in my hands, I was finding it difficult to pick things up. Even picking up a cup of tea was hard. Most of the pain was caused by the inflammation, but strange as it seems now, I didn't realise I was getting weaker. I thought all the debility was due to the pain.

The doctor couldn't or wouldn't accept that something was wrong. I knew that something was seriously wrong with my health but even if I had been able to afford to go to a private doctor, I wouldn't have known where to go. To assume it was arthritis or rheumatism or what? My mother had died with

Parkinson's disease and I know that she had pains in the joints; this was a fear in my mind that I had the same thing. I have learned since that Parkinson's is not an autoimmune illness and I have no worries in that area.

We trust our doctors implicitly but they don't know everything. I think many don't like to admit this, it appears to be a case of: "If I don't know what your illness is, then you are not ill." I have since spoken to others and they have had similar experiences. Some people even struggle for more years than I did.

The turning point came when I had the second operation for carpal tunnel syndrome. I told the surgeon some of the problems I had been having and about the pain in my hands. He looked at my fingers which were fat and swollen and hardly able to bend. He mentioned the shiny skin and said this could be a sign of something; he didn't want to make me anxious so he said it didn't have to mean it was serious but he would refer me to a rheumatologist. A month later I had an appointment with a specialist. I think he must have put in a request for urgency because the health service normally takes a lot longer than this. It can take up to 18 weeks to get an appointment.

At my appointment with the rheumatologist, he looked at the skin on my neck and chest which covered quite a large area by then and was hard and itchy. It also looked red around the edges, almost as if I had been in the sun. He said it looked like Scleroderma and he tested my strength and examined me. Next day I had to go back for x-rays to my hands and chest and blood tests. They had to take 10 bottles and the nurse asked if I would like to do half and go back the next day but I said they might as well do it at once.

Two weeks later I got a diagnosis. It was Scleroderma and Polymyositis, the second disease he had not expected. This is called an "overlap" illness and it is not as bad because apparently anyone who gets both gets a milder form of each.

He started me on a dose of 40mg of Prednisolone daily, a steroid. Apparently, the withered arms and legs were muscle loss caused by the Polymyositis, which is inflammation of the muscles. The x-rays to my hands had not shown any deformities and he told me I did not have arthritis. I had an echocardiogram, lung function tests and a DXA scan for Osteoporosis. The echocardiogram showed weakness of the heart caused by the muscle weakness. The DXA showed only a six percent possibility of getting Osteoporosis in the next twenty years. So it is not likely that I will develop it, which is something about which I am happy.

When I got home on that day I took the first dose of Prednisolone but didn't notice any change during the day. In the night I had to get up, so I sat on the edge of the bed as usual trying to get the courage to stand up. When I did there was no pain. I couldn't believe it. It was like a miracle. After more than eight months of being almost debilitated and then to have no pain is difficult to describe. The pain hadn't completely disappeared but the terrible feeling of all my tendons being stretched had just about gone. I still had a lot of difficulty walking and stiffness but the steroids stopped the swelling of my legs and hands within weeks. It was the swelling which had been the cause of a lot of the pain. For so long I had not been able to bend my legs and slowly it was improving.

Even though it was not easy, and I was always fatigued, I forced myself to walk everywhere. After ten months of taking the medicine I could again walk normally.

I was told the steroids would cause weight gain and I talked to someone I knew who had put on a lot of weight with them. The steroids did make me feel very hungry and whenever I had hunger pangs I would eat fruit or wholemeal bread. A new bakery had opened in town which sold very tasty wholemeal bread and I almost lived on bread and butter. I would have one main meal a day and then fruit and bread most of the rest of the day. I only put back on the five kilos I had lost and I am sure all the walking had a lot to do with this too. I noticed my arms were looking very nice and not old anymore. For the first few weeks of taking steroids, I would have dizzy spells in the morning shortly after taking my medicine. I also developed a "moon face". My nephew said it looked like hamster cheeks. As I got stronger and the pain got less the doctor slowly reduced the dosage until a year later I was on 1 mg every other day. In July 2012 they were stopped altogether. By then my face seemed to be almost back to normal and the double chins had gone.

A month after the diagnosis, at the beginning of May 2011, I went back to the doctor and he started me on a course of Mycophenolate Mofetil. This medicine is used after organ transplants but it has been found useful for diseases like Scleroderma and Psoriasis. For the first month of taking the steroids my energy level went up and I was sleeping better. When I started on the Mycophenolate I noticed immediately that I was always tired and my new found energy seemed to have gone.

After a couple of months the doctor said my strength was back to normal but that the fatigue would take a lot longer to overcome. Almost every day since I first started on the medication I would walk for at least an hour even though at the beginning it was a great struggle. I would even count my steps or look for landmarks, such as a monkey puzzle tree in someone's garden. The town centre is about 20 minutes' walk from my house but in those days it would take double that time. Luckily, there are plenty of places to sit along the way.

In the beginning I had to see the doctor every month and have blood tests monthly too. I was referred to Professor Denton at the Royal Free Hospital in London and received an appointment in October 2011. Professor Denton is considered by everyone who sees him to be the best. I went with a list of questions and he dealt with everything on my list without me having to ask. He recommended that I take the Mycophenolate for another 2 years. He also said I could see him regularly instead of my own doctor in the hospital if I wanted to. I am very satisfied with the treatment from my doctor in the hospital in Ipswich in Suffolk and told him I was happy to stay with him. He mentioned that I might be referred to London again if my doctor thought it was necessary.

On the same day I had routine blood tests and a nail fold capillary test. This is to test how much the hands have been affected by the Raynaud's. I saw a different doctor for this; he put a drop of oil on the skin at the base of my fingernails. Then he examined them under a microscope to look for abnormalities in the blood vessels which are called capillaries. As I had not had Raynaud's for very long, only a few of them were deformed.

He also did a thermography test. This entailed putting my hands in icy water until they were very cold and then looking at them on the thermal imager and waiting to see how long they took to warm up. The cold areas looked black and at the end only one finger of my right hand still looked black. This finger is usually the first one to go completely white when my hands are cold. If my fingers stay white for more than a few minutes, then when they eventually warm up, they can be painful for many hours afterwards, even a day or more.

I had an appointment with Professor Denton's specialist nurse who gave me some useful information and leaflets. The most useful has been one with exercises for my face; the ones I make sure I always do are the ones to stretch my mouth. One of the problems with Scleroderma is that it causes the mouth to

21

shrink. Some peoples' mouth shrinks so much it is impossible to clean their teeth properly or get dental work done. After regularly working on the exercises I have been able to increase the width of my mouth opening from 30mm at its worst to 55mm. This is a great improvement and I think my mouth is back to normal but I make sure I keep up the exercises or my mouth begins to feel tight and stiff. There were free samples of creams which I picked up. The best one I found was Doublebase Gel, it stops the skin itching and keeps my face, chest and hands soft. I use it all the time now.

I feel better now than I have for a long time but I still get fatigued. I notice it more when I am hungry and a small snack makes a big difference. In March 2012 I returned to work and thought it would be very hard but at the beginning it was fine, though after the first few months the fatigue started again. I work four days a week now and that helps but when the weather is cold I am more tired. I suppose my body is using all my energy to keep warm and that causes the excessive tiredness. This is a common complaint but the only thing is not to overdo things. I find that on the days I work I don't have much energy to go out anywhere but on my days off then my energy levels are much higher. In the cold weather I find it harder to do much but as the weather is warming up it is better.

My rheumatologist is a specialist and researcher in vasculitis and a lecturer at the university in Ipswich. Vasculitis is an autoimmune illness which has some symptoms similar to Scleroderma. On one of my appointments he asked my permission to send my notes to Oxford University where they are doing research into this disease.

I told him about my research online into my symptoms the year before I saw him and that I had come up with the same diagnosis that he gave me. He did not laugh but said that there is a lot of information to be found online. I told him that I go onto the forum of the Raynaud's and Scleroderma Association and that I had received useful information from other members of the forum. He said these forums are very good and that some of the people on them know more than the doctors.

Now that my illness is controlled and I know more about it, I realise that I am luckier than a lot of people. Except for the fatigue, which I can control by not overdoing things, I don't actually have many problems now. I sometimes have pain in my knees and of course the Raynaud's in my hands and feet but I as long as I keep warm, it is not a problem. If the hands are cold for too long then digital ulcers can form. I have not had these, but one day I did get a pitted scar on one of my fingertips. It was painful and lasted for a few weeks. I make sure I keep my hands as dry as possible and well moisturized with Doublebase.

During the time I was waiting to find out the reason for my pain and suffering, I thought it would never end. Now, it doesn't seem possible that I went through it all.

There are different forms of Scleroderma, mine is diffuse cutaneous systemic sclerosis which means it covers the whole body. Another doctor in my surgery that I saw for something unrelated told me that the symptoms of Scleroderma are not immediately apparent in my face. It is the changes in the face which can cause most distress because of the disfigurement.

Online research

During the time I was researching my symptoms online, I found that many people were doing exactly the same thing. I discovered forums for all kinds of ailments and that a lot of desperate people are being failed by the medical systems all over the world.

I couldn't understand why so many people could not get any kind of satisfactory answer from their doctors. I have since learned that because of the similarity of the symptoms between different diseases doctors often don't know what they are looking at. They don't know what tests to order.

If a patient complains of debilitating pain and the symptoms appear to indicate severe arthritis, when the doctor examines the patient and sees no abnormalities in bones, then he doesn't know what to recommend. There is often a tendency for a doctor to think the illness is imaginary and there might be something else affecting the patient, like depression, for example.

In the UK because the NHS is running out of funds and cuts are being made, doctors are told not to order blood tests unless the circumstances are dire. Blood tests are needed to diagnose auto immune diseases and so the cut backs often mean that patients suffer in pain until they are almost crippled.

This is a state of affairs which does not need to exist. It is my opinion that these online resources could be used to help people who cannot get any help from their own GP. After a certain time of trying to get a diagnosis, it would be a good idea if there was a way to register online with a health service where it is possible to give all the symptoms which are being experienced. Then specialists could give an appointment to see the patient, bypassing the GP.

The system now is that to be referred to a specialist a GP must have an idea of what the illness is, that the patient is suffering. If he cannot recognise the symptoms then he does not know which department the patient needs to be referred to, ending up with longer suffering because of non-referral.

If it is possible for the layman to diagnose himself from putting his symptoms into Google, then it should be possible to find the right doctor. A doctor who specialises in Scleroderma, for example, recognises the symptoms when he sees them. I have spoken to several people on forums who have found out their illness by putting the symptoms into Google just as I did. When they were finally diagnosed it was a relief to them, just as it was to me.

I know it is impossible to expect a general practitioner to know all illnesses, they generally deal with the same things year in, year out, but that is no help to someone desperate to find out about their health problem.

The Internet is one of the most important developments in modern times and it can and should be used much more than it is.

Links to information about Scleroderma

When I was diagnosed with Scleroderma, the doctor did not say much about it except to say that it was an autoimmune disease. I picked up a leaflet from the hospital which was printed by the Arthritis Research Campaign which gave a little information and I looked on their website.

I spent a lot of time researching Scleroderma and Polymyositis during the first months after my diagnosis. There is a lot of information online and there are several forums comprised of people with various autoimmune diseases. My favourite one is HealthUnlocked which is from the Raynaud's and Scleroderma Association, the link for the forum is:

http://raynauds.healthunlocked.com/

The Scleroderma Society has a forum at:

http://www.sclero.org/forums/forum/17-scleroderma-society-uk/

It is not necessary to be a member of the Society or Association to be a member of the forum. Anyone from any part of the world can join and I found it very helpful to read what other people were going through and ask questions, I sometimes have been able to give helpful hints to others on where to get facial exercises for example or which creams I have found the best for the skin. All these little things help and it takes away the feeling of hopelessness which many find at the beginning because of the general lack of knowledge of this disease.

Some more links:

http://www.arthritisresearchuk.org/arthritis-information/conditions/scleroderma.aspx

http://www.nhs.uk/conditions/scleroderma/Pages/Introduction.aspx

http://www.sclerodermasociety.co.uk/

http://www.scleroderma.org.uk/

http://www.fesca-scleroderma.eu/

http://www.raynauds.org.uk/

http://www.umm.edu/patiented/articles/what_symptoms_of_scleroderma_000088_2.htm

http://www.sclerodermaaustralia.com.au/

If you are lucky enough to have a rheumatologist who refers you to see Professor Denton or one of his team at the Royal Free Hospital in London then you will know you are good hands. Professor Denton is one of the most knowledgeable doctors on Scleroderma and related illnesses. He heads a research programme into the disease. He is respected by all his patients as he looks at each one as a human being and not just another name on his list.

I saw him in October 2011 and he was very thorough and covered everything that I wanted to discuss without me having to tell him. I had a list ready and when I referred to it, I had nothing extra to ask him. He gave me the option of travelling to London to see him rather than my own rheumatologist but I am happy with the care I receive. He made recommendations to my doctor who followed them and my medication is to be reviewed in October this year. (2013)

His specialist nurse gave me leaflets on maintaining facial mobility through exercise, hand exercises and one on hand waxing to relieve tight, painful skin and painful joints. They also had a selection of creams and salves for the skin, free for patients to take. They were all good but the one I use all the time now is Doublebase gel. I get it on prescription from the doctor.

The nursing team at the Royal Free Hospital is always available for patients to telephone and get advice. If you are not a patient with the hospital it might still be possible to get information and help. Following is the link for the Royal Free:

http://www.royalfree.nhs.uk/

The following link gives some information into the background of Professor Denton. He is one of a team of excellent doctors.

http://www.eustar.org/index.php?module=ContentExpress&func=display&ceid=83

In many countries research is being done into Scleroderma and there is a lot of information to be found for anyone suffering from this disease. As I was always healthy I used not to have much sympathy for others' ailments, but now realise aches and pains and tiredness are not excuses for lazy people. They can often be a very serious illness and because the person does not look sick, does not mean that they are not. Since being ill I seem to notice whether people look healthy or not, it is as if my eyes have been opened to something new.

I think that there should be training for GPs to make them more aware of the symptoms of auto immune illnesses. I am not the only one who has visited the doctor for several months, knowing something was wrong and being told that taking painkillers should sort out the problem in a few weeks.

Endnote:

I hope this small book is helpful and gives some useful information about Scleroderma. The forums are very good and I recommend them.

The most important thing for someone who has been diagnosed with Scleroderma is to have hope and determination to get better. I was determined not to succumb to it and I think that has as much to do with my recovery as the treatment.

www.ingramcontent.com/pod-product-compliance
Lightning Source LLC
Chambersburg PA
CBHW070934290526
45795CB00003B/1022